ATKINS DIET"

THE WEIGHT WATCHERS THERAPY

The wholesome yum of eating
healthy and beating obesity

KIMBERLY HOMOLKA

INTRODUCTION

A healthy weight is a significant component of good wellbeing. The amount you eat—and what you eat—assume focal jobs in keeping up a solid weight or shedding pounds. Exercise is the other key entertainer.

For quite a long time, low-fat eating regimens were believed to be the most ideal approach to shed pounds. A developing assemblage of proof shows that low-fat counts calories frequently don't work, to some degree in light of the fact that these weight control plans regularly supplant fat with effectively processed sugars. Eating a well-adjusted eating routine can assist you with getting the calories and supplements you have to fuel your every day exercises, including customary exercise.

With regards to eating nourishments to fuel your activity execution, it's not as straightforward as picking vegetables over doughnuts. You have to eat the correct kinds of nourishment at the correct occasions of the day.

Find out about the significance of sound morning meals, exercise bites, and dinner plans.

TABLE OF CONTENTS

CHAPTER ONE 1

WATCH YOUR WEIGHT 1

HOW WOULD I KNOW WHETHER I'M AT A SOLID WEIGHT? 2

WHAT CAN LOOSING WEIGHT ACCOMPLISH FOR ME? 4

MAKE A MOVE: SET GOALS 5

KEEP A NOURISHMENT AND MOVEMENT JOURNAL. 6

GET PROGRESSIVELY PHYSICAL ACTION. 7

CHAPTER TWO 9

STAYING ACTIVE AT ANY SIZE 9

WHY SHOULD I BE ACTIVE 9

FOR WHAT REASON WOULD IT BE A GOOD IDEA FOR ME TO BE DYNAMIC? 11

WHAT DO I HAVE TO THINK ABOUT BECOMING ACTIVE? 14

HERE ARE A FEW HINTS FOR STAYING SAFE DURING PHYSICAL ACTION: 16

WHAT SORTS OF EXERCISES WOULD I BE ABLE TO DO? 18

STROLLING 19

DANCING..21

BICYCLING 22

WATER EXERCISES 24

STRENGHT TRAINING...................................28

MIND AND BODY WORK OUT.......................31

DAY BY DAY LIFE EXERCISES 33

WHERE CAN I BE ACTIVE? 34

TIPS FOR PICKING A WELLNESS CENTER 35

HOW CAN I STICK WITH MY PHYSICAL ACTIVITY PLAN?..36

CHAPTER THREE 42

DIETING AND WEIGHT LOSS.........................42

1. IRREGULAR FASTING 43

2. PLANT-BASED WEIGHT CONTROL PLANS.47

3. LOW-CARB SLIMS DOWN 52

4. THE PALEO DIET 56

5. LOW-FAT SLIMS DOWN............................59

CHAPTER ONE

WATCH YOUR WEIGHT

The Basics: Overview

To remain at a sound weight, balance the calories you eat and drink with the calories you consume (go through). Calories are a proportion of the vitality in the nourishments you eat. To shed pounds, you have to consume a greater number of calories than you eat.

A sound diet and physical movement can assist you with controlling your weight. You consume more calories when you are physically dynamic.

HOW WOULD I KNOW WHETHER I'M AT A SOLID WEIGHT?

Discovering your Body Mass Index (BMI) is a simple method to learn in the event that you are at a sound weight. Utilize this Body Mass Index (BMI) adding machine to discover your BMI and what it implies for you.

In the event that you are overweight and have hazard factors for coronary illness (like hypertension or elevated cholesterol), or in the event that you have heftiness, attempt to get thinner. You can get more fit by eating less calories and getting increasingly physical movement.

In the event that you are at a sound weight, find a way to remain at a similar weight. You can remain at a similar load by getting customary physical movement and eating the correct number of calories.

In the event that you figure you may be underweight, converse with your primary care physician or medical caretaker about how to put on weight in a sound way.

How would I know whether I'm eating the correct number of calories?

Utilize the My Plate Plan to get a thought of what number of calories you have to keep up your present weight.

In the event that your weight remains the equivalent for a while, you are eating the correct number of calories to keep up your weight.

To get thinner, take a stab at eating 500 to 750 less calories every day

WHAT CAN LOOSING WEIGHT ACCOMPLISH FOR ME?

Being overweight or having heftiness can raise your hazard for genuine wellbeing conditions like:

Type 2 diabetes

Coronary illness

Hypertension

Getting in shape can:

Lower your circulatory strain

Lower your glucose

Raise your HDL (great) cholesterol

Lower your LDL (awful) cholesterol

You may begin to see these medical advantages by losing only 5 to 10 percent of your body weight. For instance, on the off chance that you weigh 200 pounds, this would mean losing 10 to 20 pounds.

MAKE A MOVE: SET GOALS
Start by making a guarantee to eat well, move more, and get support from loved ones.

SET PRACTICAL OBJECTIVES.

In the event that you have to get in shape, do it gradually after some time. Begin by defining little objectives, as:

I need to lose 1 to 2 pounds every week.

I will begin by including 10 minutes of physical action to my every day schedule.

I will curtail second helpings of dinners.

KEEP A NOURISHMENT AND MOVEMENT JOURNAL.
At the point when you know your propensities, it's simpler to make changes. Record:

What you eat

At the point when you eat

Where you eat

The amount you eat

Your physical action

How you are feeling

GET PROGRESSIVELY PHYSICAL ACTION.
Keep in mind that to shed pounds, you have to consume a bigger number of calories than you eat. Get dynamic to adjust the calories you take in with the calories you use.

Go for at any rate 2 hours and 30 minutes of vigorous physical movement seven days. For instance, take a stab at taking a lively walk.

Attempt to do oxygen consuming action for 30 minutes 5 times each week.

Do muscle-fortifying exercises two times per week. Have a go at lifting loads or doing push-ups.

Indeed, even some physical action is superior to none. On the off chance that you don't possess energy for 30 minutes of action, get going for shorter 10-minute time spans for the duration of the day.

How much action you need will rely upon your weight objectives. You may need to complete 5 hours of moderate-force action seven days to meet your objectives.

CHAPTER TWO

STAYING ACTIVE AT ANY SIZE

Physical action may appear to be hard in case you're overweight. You may get shy of breath or tired rapidly. Finding or managing the correct garments and hardware might be disappointing. Or then again, maybe you may not get a handle on happy with working before others.

The uplifting news is you can defeat these difficulties. Not exclusively would you be able to be dynamic at any size, you can have a ton of fun and feel great simultaneously.

WHY SHOULD I BE ACTIVE

Research emphatically shows that physical action is alright for nearly everybody. The medical advantages of physical movement far exceed the risks.

The exercises talked about here are alright for the vast majority. On the off chance that you have issues moving or remaining unfaltering on your feet, or in the event that you escape breath effectively, chat with a medicinal services proficient before you start. You additionally should chat with a medicinal services proficient in the event that you are uncertain of your wellbeing, have any worries that physical action might be perilous for you, or have a ceaseless illness, for example, diabetes, hypertension, or coronary illness a bone or joint issue—for instance, in your back, knee, or hip—that could deteriorate on the off chance that you change your physical movement level

FOR WHAT REASON WOULD IT BE A GOOD IDEA FOR ME TO BE DYNAMIC?

Being dynamic may assist you with living longer and shield you from creating genuine medical issues, for example, type 2 diabetes, coronary illness, stroke, and particular sorts of malignancy NIH outside connection. Ordinary physical movement is connected to numerous medical advantages, for example, lower circulatory strain and blood glucose, or glucose solid bones, muscles, and joints a solid heart and lungs better rest around evening time and improved temperament

The Physical Activity Guidelines for Americans, second version External connection (PDF, 14.2 MB), characterize standard physical action as in any event 150 minutes per seven day stretch of moderate-power high-impact movement, for example, energetic strolling. Energetic strolling is a pace of 3 miles for each hour or quicker. A moderate-force movement causes you to inhale more earnestly yet doesn't exhaust or overheat you. You ought to likewise muscle-reinforcing exercises at any rate 2 days per week.

You may arrive at this objective by beginning with 5 minutes of physical action a few times each day, 5 to 6 days every week. You could then bit by bit work as long as 10 minutes for every session, 3 times each day. On the off chance that you do significantly greater movement, you may increase considerably more wellbeing benefits.

At the point when joined with good dieting, ordinary physical action may likewise assist you with controlling your weight. In any case, examine shows that regardless of whether you can't shed pounds or keep up your weight reduction, despite everything you can appreciate significant medical advantages from ordinary physical activity.

Physical action additionally can be a great deal of fun on the off chance that you do exercises you appreciate and are dynamic with other individuals. Being dynamic with others may allow you to meet new individuals or invest more energy with loved ones. You additionally may move and inspire each other to get and remain dynamic.

WHAT DO I HAVE TO THINK ABOUT BECOMING ACTIVE?

Picking physical exercises that match your wellness level and wellbeing objectives can assist you with remaining roused and shield you from getting hurt.[1] You may feel some minor distress or muscle irritation when you previously become dynamic. These sentiments ought to leave as you become accustomed to your movement. Be that as it may, on the off chance that you feel wiped out to your stomach or have torment, you may have done excessively. Go simpler and afterward gradually develop your action level. A few exercises, for example, strolling or water exercises, are more averse to cause wounds.

In the event that you have been dormant, start gradually and perceive how you feel. Progressively increment to what extent and how frequently you are dynamic. On the off chance that you need direction, check with a medicinal services or guaranteed wellness proficient.

HERE ARE A FEW HINTS FOR STAYING SAFE DURING PHYSICAL ACTION:

Wear the correct security gear, for example, a bicycle head protector on the off chance that you are bicycling.

Ensure any athletic gear you use works and fits appropriately.

Search for safe spots to be dynamic. For example, stroll in sufficiently bright territories where other individuals are near. Be dynamic with a companion or gathering.

Remain hydrated to supplant the body liquids you lose through perspiring and to keep you from getting overheated.

In the event that you are dynamic outside, shield yourself from the sun with sunscreen and a cap or defensive visor and garments.

Wear enough attire to keep warm in cold or breezy climate. Layers are ideal.

On the off chance that you don't feel right, stop your movement. In the event that you have any of the accompanying notice signs, stop and look for help immediately:

Agony, snugness, or weight in your chest or neck, shoulder, or arm Outrageous brevity of breath, unsteadiness or disorder

Check with a medicinal services proficient about what to do on the off chance that you have any of these notice signs. On the off chance that your action is causing torment in your joints, feet, lower legs, or legs, you additionally ought to counsel a social insurance expert to check whether you may need to change the sort or measure of movement you are doing.

WHAT SORTS OF EXERCISES WOULD I BE ABLE TO DO?
You don't should be a competitor or have unique aptitudes or hardware to make physical action some portion of your life. Numerous sorts of exercises you do each day, for example, strolling your canine or going all over strides at home or at work, may help improve your wellbeing.

Attempt various exercises you appreciate. On the off chance that you like an action, you're bound to stay with it. Anything that makes you move around, in any event, for a couple of moments one after another, is a sound beginning to getting fit.

STROLLING
Strolling is free and simple to do—and you can do it anyplace. Strolling will support you

Burn calories

Improve your wellness

Lift your state of mind

Fortify your bones and muscles

On the off chance that you are worried about security, take a stab at strolling in a shopping center or park where it is sufficiently bright and other individuals are near. Numerous shopping centers and stops have seats where you can take a snappy break. Strolling with a companion or relative is more secure than strolling alone and may give the social help you have to meet your action objectives.

In the event that you don't possess energy for a long walk, go for a few short strolls. For instance, rather than a 30-minute walk, add three 10-minute strolls to your day. Shorter spurts of movement are simpler to fit into a bustling timetable.

STROLLING TIPS

Wear agreeable, well-fitting strolling shoes with a ton of help, and socks that ingest sweat.

Dress for the climate in the event that you are strolling outside. In chilly climate, wear layers of apparel you can evacuate in the event that you start getting excessively warm. In sweltering climate, secure yourself against the sun and warmth.

Warm up by strolling all the more gradually for the initial few moments. Chill off by easing back your pace.

DANCING
Dancing can be a great deal of fun while it conditions your muscles,

fortifies your heart and lungs, and lifts your state of mind. You can move at a fitness center, move studio, or even at home. Simply turn on some enthusiastic music and start moving. You likewise can move to a video on your TV or PC.

On the off chance that you experience difficulty remaining on your feet for quite a while, take a stab at moving while at the same time plunking down. Seat moving gives you a chance to move your arms and legs to music while dropping the weight from your feet.

BICYCLING
Riding a bike spreads your weight among your arms, back, and hips. For open air biking, you might need to attempt an off-road bicycle. Trail

blazing bicycles have more extensive tires and are sturdier than bicycles with more slender tires. You can purchase a bigger seat to make biking progressively agreeable.

For indoor biking, you might need to attempt a prostrate bicycle. On this kind of bicycle, you sit lower to the ground with your legs coming to advance to the pedals. Your body is in even more a leaning back position, which may feel superior to sitting straight up. The seat on a supine bicycle is likewise more extensive than the seat on a normal bicycle.

On the off chance that you choose to purchase a bicycle, check how much weight it can support to ensure it is alright for you.

EXERCISE GARMENTS TIPS

Garments made of textures that retain sweat are best for working out.

Agreeable, lightweight garments enable you to move all the more effectively.

Tights or spandex shorts are the best bottoms to wear to avoid inward thigh abrading.

Ladies should wear a bra that gives additional help during physical action.

WATER EXERCISES
Swimming and water exercises put less weight on your joints than strolling, moving, or biking. In the event that your feet, back, or joints hurt when you stand, water

exercises might be best for you. In the event that you feel reluctant about wearing a swimming outfit, you can wear shorts and a T-shirt while you swim.

PRACTICING IN WATER

gives you a chance to be increasingly adaptable. You can move your body in water in manners you will be unable to ashore.

diminishes your danger of harming yourself. Water gives a characteristic pad, which shields you from beating or shaking your joints.

Averts sore muscles.

Keeps you cool, in any event, when you are buckling down.

You don't have to realize how to swim to turn out in water. You can do shallow-or profound water practices at either end of the pool without swimming. For example, you can do laps while clutching a kickboard and kicking your feet. You additionally can walk or run over the width of the pool while moving your arms.

For shallow-water exercises, the water level ought to be between your midsection and chest. During profound water exercises, the greater part of your body is submerged. For security and solace, wear a froth belt or life coat.

TIPS FOR PROTECTING YOUR HAIR

In case you're stressed that pool water will harm or wreckage up your hair, attempt these tips:

Utilize a dip top to help shield your hair from pool synthetic compounds and getting wet.

Wear a characteristic haircut, short meshes, locks, or turns, which might be simpler to style after a water exercise.

Purchase a cleanser to expel chlorine development, accessible at most medication stores, if your hair feels dry or harmed after a pool exercise.

STRENGHT TRAINING

Strength training includes utilizing free loads, weightlifting machines, opposition groups, or your very own body weight to make your muscles more grounded. Lower-body quality preparing will improve your parity and anticipate falls.

Strength training may support you

Construct and keep up solid muscles as you get more seasoned

keep on performing exercises of day by day living, for example, conveying food supplies or moving furnishings

Keep your bones solid, which may help anticipate osteoporosis NIH outside connection and breaks

In the event that you are simply beginning, utilizing a weightlifting machine might be more secure than hand weights. As you get fit, you might need to include free-weight practices with hand weights.

You needn't bother with a weight seat or enormous hand weights to do quality preparing at home. You can utilize a couple of hand loads to do bicep twists. You can likewise utilize your own body weight: for instance, get here and there from a seat.

Legitimate structure is significant when lifting loads. You may hurt yourself on the off chance that you don't lift loads appropriately. You might need to plan a session with an affirmed wellness expert to realize which activities to do and how to do them securely. Check with your wellbeing back up plan about whether your wellbeing plan covers these administrations.

On the off chance that you choose to purchase a home rec center, check how much weight it can support to ensure it is ok for you.

STRENGTH TRAINING TIPS

Go for at any rate 2 days out of each seven day stretch of reinforce preparing exercises.

Attempt to play out each activity 8 to multiple times. In the event that that is excessively hard, the weight you are lifting is excessively overwhelming. On the off chance that it's excessively simple, your weight is excessively light.

Attempt to practice all the significant muscle gatherings. These gatherings incorporate the muscles of the legs, hips, chest, back, mid-region, shoulders, and arms.

Try not to work similar muscles 2 days straight. Your muscles need time to recuperate.

MIND AND BODY WORK OUT
Your nearby medical clinic or wellness, amusement, or public venue may offer classes, for example, yoga, jujitsu, or Pilates. You additionally may discover a portion of these exercises on the web and can download them to a PC, advanced cell, or other gadget.

These kinds of exercises may support you

become more grounded and increasingly adaptable

feel increasingly loose

improve equalization and stance

These classes additionally can be a great deal of fun and change up your exercise schedule. In the event that a few developments are difficult to do or you have wounds you are worried about, converse with the educator about how to adjust the activities and postures to address your issues—or start with a tenderfoot's class.

DAY BY DAY LIFE EXERCISES

Day by day life exercises, for example, clearing out the storage room or washing the vehicle, are incredible approaches to get going. Little changes can add progressively physical movement to your day and improve your wellbeing. Attempt these:

Take 2-to 3-minute strolling breaks at work a few times each day, if conceivable.

Stand, walk, or stretch set up during TV ads.

Take the stairs rather than the lift or elevator at whatever point you can.

Park more distant from where you are proceeding to walk the remainder of the way.

Indeed, even a shopping excursion can be practice since it gives an opportunity to walk and convey your packs. Tasks, for example, cutting the yard, raking leaves, and planting additionally check.

WHERE CAN I BE ACTIVE?
You can see numerous fun places as dynamic. Having more than one spot may shield you from getting exhausted. Here are a few alternatives:

Join or take a class at a neighborhood wellness, amusement, or public venue.

Appreciate the outside by clearing out or taking a stroll in a protected nearby park, neighborhood, or shopping center.

Work out in the solace of your own home with an exercise video or by finding a wellness channel on your TV, tablet, or other cell phone.

TIPS FOR PICKING A WELLNESS CENTER

Ensure the middle has practice hardware for individuals who gauge more and staff to tell you the best way to utilize it.

Inquire as to whether the middle has any unique classes for individuals simply beginning, more established grown-ups, or individuals with versatility or medical problems.

Check whether you can evaluate the middle or take a class before you join.

Attempt to locate an inside near work or home. The snappier and simpler the middle is to get to, the better your odds of utilizing it regularly.

Ensure you comprehend the standards for joining and consummation your enrollment, what your participation charge covers, any related expenses, and the days and long periods of activity.

HOW CAN I STICK WITH MY PHYSICAL ACTIVITY PLAN?

Sticking with a plan to be physically active can be a challenge. Online tools such as the NIH Body Weight Planner can help. The NIH Body Weight Planner lets you tailor your calorie and physical activity plans to reach your personal goals within a specific time period.

A person tying their running shoes while wearing a fitness tracker band

Devices you can wear, such as pedometers and fitness trackers, may help you count steps, calories, and minutes of physical activity.

You also can download fitness apps that let you enter information to track your progress using a computer or smart phone or other mobile device.

Devices you can wear, such as pedometers and fitness trackers, may help you count steps, calories, and minutes of physical activity. Trackers can help you set goals and monitor progress. You wear most of these devices on your wrist like a watch, or clipped to your clothing.

Keeping an activity journal is another good way to help you stay motivated and on track to reach your fitness goals.

SET GOALS. As you track your activity, try to set specific short- and long-term goals. For example, instead of "I will be more active," set a goal such as "I will take a walk after lunch at least 2 days a week." Getting started with a doable goal is a good way to form a new habit. A short-term goal may be to walk 5 to 10 minutes, 5 days a week. A long-term goal may be to do at least 150 minutes of moderate-intensity physical activity a week.

GET SUPPORT. Ask a family member or friend to be active with you. Your workout buddy can help make your activities more fun and can cheer you on and help you meet your goals.

TRACK PROGRESS. You may not feel as though you are making progress, but when you look back at where you started, you may be pleasantly surprised. Making regular activity part of your life is a big step. Start slowly and praise yourself for every goal you set and achieve.

REVIEW YOUR GOALS. Did you meet your goals? If not, why? Are they doable? Did you hit a roadblock trying to meet your goal? What will you do differently next week? Brainstorm some options to overcome future roadblocks. Ask a friend or family member to help support your goals.

PICK NONFOOD REWARDS. Whether your goal is to be active 15 minutes a day, to walk farther than you did last week, or simply to stay positive, recognizing your efforts is an important part of staying on track. Decide how you will reward yourself. Some ideas for rewards include getting new music to charge you up or buying new workout gear.

BE PATIENT WITH YOURSELF. Don't get discouraged if you have setbacks from time to time. If you can't achieve your goal the first time or can only stick to your goals for part of the week, remind yourself that this is all part of establishing new habits.

LOOK AHEAD. Try to focus on what you will do differently moving forward, rather than on what went wrong. Pat yourself on the back for trying.

MOST IMPORTANTLY, DON'T GIVE UP. Any movement, even for a short time, is a good thing. Each activity you add to your life is another step toward a healthier you.

CHAPTER THREE

DIETING AND WEIGHT LOSS

The 8 Best Diet Plans — Sustainability, Weight Loss, and the sky is the limit from there

It's evaluated that almost 50% of American grown-ups endeavor to get in shape every year (1Trusted Source).

Probably the most ideal approaches to shed pounds is by changing your eating routine.

However, the sheer number of accessible eating regimen plans may make it hard to begin, as you're uncertain which one is most appropriate, feasible, and compelling.

A few eats less carbs mean to control your craving to lessen your nourishment admission, while others recommend limiting your admission of calories and either carbs or fat.

In addition, many offer medical advantages that go past weight reduction.

Here are the 8 best diet intends to assist you with shedding weight and improve your general wellbeing.

1. IRREGULAR FASTING
Irregular fasting is a dietary system that cycles between times of fasting and eating.

Different structures exist, including the 16/8 technique, which includes constraining your calorie admission to 8 hours out of every day, and the 5:2 strategy, which confines your day by day calorie admission to 500–600 calories two times seven days.

How it functions: Intermittent fasting limits the time you're permitted to eat, which is a straightforward method to lessen your calorie consumption. This can prompt weight reduction — except if you remunerate by eating a lot of nourishment during permitted eating periods.

Weight reduction: In a survey of studies, discontinuous fasting was appeared to cause 3–8% weight reduction more than 3–24 weeks, which is a fundamentally more prominent rate than different techniques (2Trusted Source).

A similar survey indicated that along these lines of eating may lessen midriff perimeter by 4–7%, which is a marker for hurtful paunch fat (2Trusted Source).

Different ponders found that discontinuous fasting can build fat copying while at the same time safeguarding bulk, which can improve digestion (3Trusted Source, 4Trusted Source).

Different benefits: Intermittent fasting has been connected to hostile to maturing impacts, expanded insulin affectability, improved cerebrum wellbeing, decreased irritation, and numerous different advantages (5Trusted Source, 6Trusted Source).

Drawbacks: all in all, irregular fasting is ok for most sound grown-ups.

All things considered, those delicate to drops in their glucose levels, for example, a few people with diabetes, low weight, or a dietary issue, just as pregnant or breastfeeding ladies, should converse with a wellbeing proficient before beginning discontinuous fasting.

Outline

Discontinuous fasting cycles between times of fasting and eating. It has been appeared to help weight reduction and is connected to numerous other medical advantages.

2. PLANT-BASED WEIGHT CONTROL PLANS

Plant-based eating regimens may assist you with getting in shape. Vegetarianism and veganism are the most famous variants, which confine creature items for wellbeing, moral, and natural reasons.

Nonetheless, increasingly adaptable plant-based consumes less calories additionally exist, for example, the flexitarian diet, which is a plant-based diet that permits eating creature items with some restraint.

How it functions: There are numerous sorts of vegetarianism, yet most include taking out all meat, poultry, and fish. A few veggie lovers may in like manner dodge eggs and dairy.

The vegetarian diet makes it a stride further by confining every single creature item, just as creature inferred items like dairy, gelatin, nectar, whey, casein, and egg whites.

There are no obvious principles for the flexitarian diet, as it's a way of life change as opposed to an eating regimen. It empowers eating generally organic products, vegetables, vegetables, and entire grains yet takes into consideration protein and creature items with some restraint, making it a famous other option.

A large number of the confined nutritional categories are high in calories, so constraining them may help weight reduction.

Weight reduction: Research shows that plant-based eating regimens are powerful for weight reduction (7Trusted Source, 8Trusted Source, 9Trusted Source).

A survey of 12 considers including 1,151 members found that individuals on a plant-based diet lost a normal of 4.4 pounds (2 kg) more than the individuals who included creature items (10Trusted Source).

Additionally, those following a veggie lover diet lost a normal of 5.5 pounds (2.5 kg) more than individuals not eating a plant-based eating routine (10Trusted Source).

Plant-based eating regimens likely guide weight reduction since they will in general be wealthy in fiber, which can assist you with remaining more full for more, and low in fatty fat (11Trusted Source, 12Trusted Source, 13Trusted Source).

Different benefits: Plant-based eats less carbs have been connected to numerous different advantages, for example, a decreased danger of incessant conditions like coronary illness, certain malignant growths, and diabetes. They can likewise be more ecologically practical than meat-based eating regimens (14Trusted Source, 15Trusted

Source, 16Trusted Source, 17Trusted Source).

Drawbacks: Though plant-based eating regimens are sound, they can limit significant supplements that are ordinarily found in creature items, for example, iron, nutrient B12, nutrient D, calcium, zinc, and omega-3 unsaturated fats.

A flexitarian approach or legitimate supplementation can help represent these supplements.

Synopsis

Plant-based eating regimens confine meat and creature items for different reasons. Studies show that they help weight reduction by diminishing your calorie admission and offer numerous different advantages.

3. LOW-CARB SLIMS DOWN
Low-carb eats less carbs are among the most mainstream abstains from food for weight reduction. Models incorporate the Atkins diet, ketogenic (keto) diet, and low-carb, high-fat (LCHF) diet.

A few assortments decrease carbs more radically than others. For example, low-carb slims down like the keto diet confine this macronutrient to under 10% of complete calories, contrasted and 30% or less for different sorts (18Trusted Source).

How it functions: Low-carb slims down limit your carb admission for protein and fat.

They're commonly higher in protein than low-fat weight control plans, which is significant, as protein can help check your hunger, raise your digestion, and save bulk (19Trusted Source, 20Trusted Source).

In low-carb consumes less calories like keto, your body starts utilizing unsaturated fats instead of carbs for vitality by changing over them into ketones. This procedure is called ketosis (21Trusted Source).

Weight reduction: Many investigations show that low-carb diets can help weight reduction and might be more viable than ordinary low-fat eating regimens (22Trusted Source, 23Trusted Source, 24Trusted Source, 25Trusted Source).

For instance, a survey of 53 examinations including 68,128 members found that low-carb counts calories brought about altogether more weight reduction than low-fat eating regimens (22Trusted Source).

Likewise, low-carb consumes less calories give off an impression of being very powerful at consuming unsafe paunch fat (26Trusted Source, 27Trusted Source, 28Trusted Source).

Different benefits: Research recommends that low-carb diets may lessen chance factors for coronary illness, including elevated cholesterol and circulatory strain levels. They may likewise improve glucose and insulin levels in individuals with type 2 diabetes (29Trusted Source, 30Trusted Source).

Drawbacks: now and again, a low-carb diet may raise LDL (terrible) cholesterol levels. Extremely low-carb diets can likewise be hard to pursue and cause stomach related miracle in certain individuals (31Trusted Source).

In uncommon circumstances, following a low-carb diet may cause a condition known as ketoacidosis, a perilous metabolic condition that can be deadly whenever left untreated (32Trusted Source, 33Trusted Source).

Synopsis

Low-carb abstains from food confine your carb admission, which urges your body to utilize increasingly fat as fuel. They can assist you with getting in shape and offer numerous different advantages.

4. THE PALEO DIET
The Paleo diet advocates eating similar nourishments that your tracker gatherer precursors purportedly ate.

It depends on the hypothesis that cutting edge sicknesses are connected toward the Western eating regimen, as advocates accept that the human body hasn't developed to process vegetables, grains, and dairy.

How it functions: The paleo diet advocates eating entire nourishments, organic products, vegetables, lean meats, nuts, and seeds. It limits the utilization of handled nourishments, grains, sugar, and dairy, however some less prohibitive variants take into account some dairy items like cheddar.

Weight reduction: Numerous investigations have demonstrated that the paleo diet can help weight reduction and decrease destructive tummy fat (34Trusted Source, 35Trusted Source, 36Trusted Source).

For instance, in one 3-week study, 14 solid grown-ups following a paleo diet lost a normal of 5.1 pounds (2.3

kg) and diminished their midriff periphery — a marker for gut fat — by a normal of 0.6 inches (1.5 cm) (37Trusted Source).

Research additionally recommends that the paleo diet might be more filling than mainstream slims down like the Mediterranean eating regimen and low-fat weight control plans. This might be because of its high protein content (38Trusted Source, 39Trusted Source).

Different benefits: Following the paleo diet may decrease a few coronary illness chance factors, for example, hypertension, cholesterol, and triglyceride levels (40Trusted Source, 41Trusted Source).

Drawbacks: Though the paleo diet is sound, it confines a few nutritious nutritional categories, including vegetables, entire grains, and dairy.

Rundown

The paleo diet advocates eating entire nourishments, comparatively to how your progenitors ate. Studies show that it might help weight reduction and diminish coronary illness hazard factors.

5. LOW-FAT SLIMS DOWN
Like low-carb slims down, low-fat abstains from food have been well known for quite a long time.

All in all, a low-fat diet includes limiting your fat admission to 30% of your every day calories.

Some very-and ultra-low-fat slims down expect to restrict fat utilization to under 10% of calories (24Trusted Source).

How it functions: Low-fat eating regimens limit fat admission since fat gives about double the quantity of calories per gram, contrasted and the other two macronutrients — protein and carbs.

Ultra-low-fat eats less contain less than 10% of calories from fat, with roughly 80% of calories originating from carbs and 10% from protein.

Ultra-low-fat abstains from food are essentially plant-based and limit meat and creature items.

Weight reduction: As low-fat eating regimens limit calorie consumption, they can help weight reduction (42Trusted Source, 43Trusted Source, 44Trusted Source, 45Trusted Source).

www.ingramcontent.com/pod-product-compliance
Lightning Source LLC
Chambersburg PA
CBHW020617220526
45463CB00006B/2611